Glenda Agra
Maria Vitoria S. Medeiros
Nilton S. Formiga

Caring for patients with neoplastic wounds

Glenda Agra
Maria Vitoria S. Medeiros
Nilton S. Formiga

Caring for patients with neoplastic wounds

the knowledge and work of nurses

ScienciaScripts

Imprint

Cover image: www.ingimage.com

This book is a translation from the original published under ISBN 978-620-2-17560-9.

Publisher:
Sciencia Scripts
is a trademark of
Dodo Books Indian Ocean Ltd. and OmniScriptum S.R.L publishing group

120 High Road, East Finchley, London, N2 9ED, United Kingdom
Str. Armeneasca 28/1, office 1, Chisinau MD-2012, Republic of Moldova, Europe
Printed at: see last page
ISBN: 978-620-7-33518-3

Table of contents:

THE KNOWLEDGE AND PRACTICE OF NURSES IN THE CARE OF

PATIENTS WITH NEOPLASTIC WOUNDS

Glenda Agra
Maria Vitoria de Souza Medeiros
Nilton Soares Formiga

SUMMARY

Neoplastic wounds represent a distressing burden for patients who face a prognosis of terminal illness, since they are lesions that have no possibility of healing, disfigure the physical appearance and develop symptoms that are difficult to control. The aim of this study was to verify the knowledge and practice of nurses in caring for patients with neoplastic wounds. This is a descriptive study with a quantitative design carried out with 22 nurses from a philanthropic hospital in Campina Grande - PB between April and June 2016. The instrument was a structured questionnaire containing questions about the care of patients with neoplastic wounds, guided by the Ministry of Health protocol. Descriptive statistics and the relevant literature were used to analyze the data. It should be noted that the research was guided by Resolution 466/2012 of the National Health Council (CNS), respecting the regulatory guidelines involving research with human beings. The results obtained allowed us, in general, to identify that nurses have gaps in their knowledge of content and techniques for assessing and treating patients with neoplastic wounds. In addition, it was found that nurses do not provide some of the care required for this clientele. In this way, the institution which was the *focus of* the research needs to invest in continuing education in order to train the nursing team to monitor patients with neoplastic lesions, acquire the necessary materials and implement care protocols to guide the practice of assessment and therapeutic methods for caring for people with neoplastic wounds, their families and caregivers.

Keywords: Knowledge. Nurses. Nursing care. Patient care. Cutaneous neoplasms.

Chapter 1

1 INTRODUCTION

Brazil is experiencing a phenomenon known as the epidemiological transition, characterized by changes in the causes of mortality and morbidity associated with demographic, social and economic transformations. In this context, chronic non-communicable diseases, including cancer, appear as one of the diseases responsible for changing the illness profile of the Brazilian population and despite advances in research and new therapeutic modalities, it is considered the second leading cause of mortality in the country.[1-2]

Cancer is defined as a genetic disease characterized by disordered cell growth and division and is therefore called a malignant tumor, which in turn can invade adjacent and/or distant tissues and organs, called metastases.[3]

Cancer estimates for Brazil for the 2016-2017 biennium indicate that there will be around 600,000 new cases of cancer; of these, approximately 180,000 new cases will be non-melanoma skin cancer. The epidemiological profile revealed that the most frequent cancers, except non-melanoma skin cancer, were prostate cancer (61,000) in men and breast cancer (58,000) in women. The most frequent types of cancer in men were prostate (28.6%), lung (8.1%), intestine (7.8%), stomach (6.0%) and oral cavity (5.2%) and in women, breast (28.1%), intestine (8.6%), cervix (7.9%), lung (5.3%) and stomach (3.7%) were among the main ones. Although there are limitations, it is believed that the estimates are capable of describing current patterns of cancer incidence, making it possible to gauge the magnitude and impact of this disease in Brazil (BRASIL, 2016). For these same years, in the Northeast region, it was estimated that there would be 47,520 new cases of cancer in men and 51,540 in women.[4]

Neoplastic wounds, also known as oncological, malignant, tumorous or fungoid lesions (when they have a mushroom or cauliflower appearance), are formed by the infiltration of malignant tumor cells into skin structures, consequently leading to a breakdown of its integrity, with the subsequent formation of an evolutionarily exophytic wound, due to the uncontrolled cell proliferation caused by the oncogenesis process.[5]

The prevalence of these lesions, regardless of anatomical location, is not well documented, but it is estimated from international studies that 5% to 10% of cancer patients develop malignant wounds.[6-7] A study carried out in Switzerland found that the prevalence of malignant lesions in patients with metastatic cancer was 6.6%.[8]

There is a lack of national epidemiological data on neoplastic wounds, so it is difficult to find reliable data on the incidence of people diagnosed with cancer who progress to developing these lesions. However, in Brazil, two recent quantitative studies have provided data on the involvement of people with malignant neoplasms, thus bringing new information that highlights the profile, characteristics and treatment of neoplastic lesions.[9-10]

The neoplastic wounds that affect the skin are yet another aggravation in the life of the cancer patient, as they progressively disfigure the body and become friable, painful, exudative and foul-smelling.[11-13] At the same time, these lesions can lead to the development of complications such as superficial and/or systemic infections, fistulas and maggot infestation; moreover, these wounds also affect the patient's psychological, social and spiritual dimensions, which can interfere with interpersonal relationships with the medical team, with family members and even socially.[6-7;14-20]

The treatment of neoplastic wounds is complex, as it requires an assessment of oncological etiology, wound characteristics, the patient's physical and emotional state and wound staging. It is therefore necessary for nurses, who are usually responsible for dressing wounds, to have the skills and ability to identify, assess and treat neoplastic wounds, providing comprehensive care for patients and their families.[21]

In order to provide a better quality of life for patients with advanced cancer and neoplastic wounds, nurses need to be familiar with specific products, substances, medicines and coverings to control signs and symptoms, as well as the economic reality of the patient, their family and the institution in which they are hospitalized, in order to better intervene.[22]

It is therefore up to the nurse to assess and treat the neoplastic lesion, taking into account the patient's physical, psychological, social, spiritual and family dimensions, in order to improve their quality of life during their last days of life, since the patient living with advanced cancer and a neoplastic wound has a high degree of physical, psychological and spiritual vulnerability.[23]

In this context, when assessing a patient with a neoplastic wound, nurses should consider the following aspects: size, depth, area of involvement, color, extent, odor, exudate, bleeding, pain, pruritus, desquamation, fistulas, abscesses, physical limitations, metastases, suitability of clothing and dressings for the patient.[24-26]

In the meantime, in 2009, the National Cancer Institute[5] (INCA) published a manual of nursing actions, of the protocol type, for patients with advanced cancer who have neoplastic wounds, with the aim of standardizing assessment and therapeutic interventions to better care for these patients.[24]

The desire to carry out this study arose from technical visits to a philanthropic hospital that treats patients with advanced cancer, where it was possible to see that the nurses were unaware of the INCA manual and often used obsolete protocols for assessing and treating wounds. It should be noted that a search was carried out in national databases using the key words "oncological wounds", "tumor wounds", "neoplastic wounds", "malignant wounds", "knowledge", "nurses" using the Boolean operators "OR" and "AND" and it was found that there were few published articles on this subject.

Based on this, the following guiding question was posed: What is the knowledge and practice of nurses in caring for patients with neoplastic wounds?

In this sense, the general objective of this study was to investigate the knowledge and practice of nurses in caring for patients with neoplastic wounds.

This research will contribute to the expansion of scientific production related to the subject, disseminating knowledge among professionals about the existence of the INCA manual and proposing, based on the data collected, a specific protocol for the care of patients with neoplastic wounds for the institution that is the *locus of* this research.

Chapter 2

2 METHODOLOGY

This is a descriptive quantitative study carried out in a philanthropic hospital in the municipality of Campiña Grande - PB. The population defined for the study was made up of nursing assistants. In order to select the sample, the following inclusion criteria were used: care nurses who performed dressings on patients with neoplastic wounds and who had at least six months' experience in the field and were carrying out their work activities on the day of collection; and exclusion criteria: nurses who were away at the time of data collection (sick leave, vacation, maternity leave or away for training). In this sense, 22 nurses from this health institution took part in the study. The sample was non-probabilistic, as we considered the subjects who, when consulted at the hospital, were willing to collaborate by answering the questionnaire presented to them by the person responsible for the research.

For data collection, a structured questionnaire was drawn up, containing two sections: the first focused on the sociodemographic and professional aspects of the research subjects, which aimed to briefly characterize the participants in this study with information on gender, age, marital status, length of academic training and length of experience in oncology and postgraduate studies. In the second part of the questionnaire, an instrument was drawn up containing questions about the care of patients with neoplastic wounds, guided by the Ministry of Health - National Cancer Institute - manual on the treatment and control of tumor wounds - MS/INCA (2011),[5] as follows:

1 - Assessment of the neoplastic wound and the patient's needs: this is an instrument made up of 17 items related to assessing the area of the lesion (e.g. location, size, staging, among others), in which the respondent indicated, respectively, their response emphasizing their **knowledge and doing of** caring for the patient who had a neoplastic wound; to **do** this, they indicated their response, regarding **knowledge, on** a three-point scale (1 = I don't know, 2 = I know in part and 3 = I know). With regard to **doing**, the same subject indicated his answers on a binomial scale (for example, 1 = yes and 2 = no).

2 - Assessment of basic neoplastic wound care: this is an instrument made up of 10 items related to assessing the area of the lesion (e.g. location, size, staging, among others), in which the respondent indicated, respectively, their response emphasizing their **knowledge and practice of** caring for a patient with a neoplastic wound; to **do** this, they indicated their response, regarding **knowledge, on** a three-point scale (1 = don't know, 2 = partly know and 3 = know). With regard to **doing**, the same subject indicated his answers on a binomial scale (for example, 1 = yes and 2 = no).

3 - Evaluation of specific tumor wound care: this

The instrument is made up of seven (7) sub-items: a) pain control, made up of 14 items; b) odor control, made up of 7 items; c) exudate control, made up of 3 items; d) bleeding control, made up of 10 items; e) necrosis control, made up of 2 items; f) skin fistula control, made up of 3 items and g) pruritus control, made up of 6 items. In all of them, the respondent indicated, respectively, his answer emphasizing his **knowledge and doing of** caring for the patient with a neoplastic wound; for this, he indicated his answer, referring to **knowledge,** on a three-point scale (1 = I don't know, 2 = I know in part and 3 = I know). With regard to **doing**, the same subject indicated his answers on a binomial scale (for example, 1 = yes and 2 = no).

4 - Recording nursing actions: this instrument consists of four (4) sub-items. In all of them, the respondent indicated, respectively, his answer emphasizing his **knowledge** and **doing of** recording information about the assessment and treatment of the patient with a neoplastic wound; to do this, he indicated his answer, regarding **knowledge, on** a three-point scale (1 = I don't know, 2 = I know in part and 3 = I know). With regard to **doing**, the same subject indicated his answers on a binomial scale (for example, 1 = yes and 2 = no).

Data was collected from May to June 2016 and descriptive statistics (mean, standard deviation and frequencies in percentages) were used to analyze the data, using the *Statistical Package for the Social Sciences* 22.0 (SPSS-22) program.

With regard to ethical considerations, this research was guided by the Code of Ethics for Nurses - Resolution No. 311/2007 of the Federal Nursing Council, as well as the Guidelines and Regulatory Norms for Research Involving Human Beings, in the

Brazilian scenario, contemplated by Resolution No. 466/2012 of the National Health Council (CNS) / Ministry of Health (MS), which deals with research with human beings.

The research project was submitted to the Research Ethics Committee (CEP) of the Alcides Carneiro University Hospital, which approved it with opinion no. 1.321.296 and CAAE no. 50354615.8.0000.5182.

Chapter 3

3 RESULTS AND DISCUSSION

Twenty-two nurses took part in the study, 91% of whom were female; 68% were married; their ages ranged from 24 to 62 years (mean = 36.6, SD = 9.31); 32% had five years of academic training; with regard to experience in the field of oncology, 54% said they had between one and two years; 14% between three and four years and 32% between five and ten years; 55% had a *lato sensu* postgraduate degree.

Once the database for this study had been collected and formatted, a frequency analysis was carried out to assess the distribution of the subjects' responses to these instruments on caring for patients with neoplastic wounds. Therefore, in order to provide a better understanding for the reader, the results will be presented in two sections: the **knowledge** and practice **of** the specific assessments highlighted in the instrument, i.e. the **knowledge** and **practice of** assessing the neoplastic wound and the patient's needs described in Table 1 will be presented first, and so on for the other assessment sections.

Table 1 - Frequency distribution of nurses' responses about **knowing** and **doing** about neoplastic wound assessment and patient needs. Campina Grande - PB, 2016.

You assess the wound and the patient's needs										
	How much do you know						How much you make			
	I don't know		I partly know		I know		Yes		No	
	F	%	F	%	F	%	F	%	F	%
1.Location	1	4	7	32	14	**64**	11	**55**	10	45
2.Size	3	14	10	**45**	9	41	8	36	13	**64**

3. staging	3	14	11	**50**	8	36	6	27	16	**73**
4. area of involvement	1	4	10	46	11	**50**	9	41	13	**59**
5.Cor	1	5	7	32	14	**64**	10	45	12	**55**
6.Extension	1	5	6	27	15	**68**	10	45	12	**55**
7.Odor	1	5	2	9	19	**86**	13	**59**	9	41
8. exudate	2	9	3	14	17	**77**	12	**56**	10	44
9. bleeding	1	5	2	9	19	**86**	12	**56**	10	44
10.Dor	1	5	2	9	19	**86**	13	**59**	9	41
H. Itching	1	5	5	23	15	**72**	10	44	12	**56**
12. decamination	3	14	7	32	12	**54**	9	41	13	**59**
13 Signs of infection	2	9	6	27	14	**64**	11	**50**	11	**50**
14.Involvement or invasion of organs or systems	5	23	7	32	10	**45**	7	32	15	**68**
15. wound progression or change	5	23	4	18	12	**59**	7	32	15	**68**

16. products needed/appropriate for the wound	4	18	9	**42**	9	40	5	23	17	**77**
17. identify the patient's or caregiver's educational needs regarding wound care after discharge	3	14	7	32	10	**54**	10	44	12	**56**
TOTAL	22	100	22	100	22	100	22	100	22	100

SOURCE: Research data, 2016

In Table 1, with regard to the **knowledge** section, it can be seen that in the majority of the items, the respondents stated that they **knew how to** assess the neoplastic wound and the patient's needs in the items: location, area of involvement, color, extent, odor, exudate, bleeding, pain, itching, scaling, signs of infection, involvement or invasion of organs or systems, progression or change of the wound and identify the educational needs of the patient or caregiver regarding wound care after discharge; on the other hand, in three items the respondents indicated that they knew how to **assess, in part, the** following items: size, staging and products needed/appropriate for the wound.

With regard to the **doing** section, the majority of the subjects answered that they **did not** assess the neoplastic wound and the patient's needs in terms of the following items: size, staging, area of involvement, color, extent, itching, scaling, signs of infection, involvement or invasion of organs or systems, progression of the wound, products needed/appropriate for the wound, identifying the educational needs of the patient or caregiver regarding wound care after discharge, and five mentioned that they **did** assess the wound on the items: location, odor, exudate, bleeding, pain and signs of infection. In this section, it is worth noting that, of all the items in the instrument, the **'signs of infection' score** was very equal, resulting in a dubious reflection on the frequency.

In the specific area of care for people with neoplastic wounds, it is essential that health professionals, including nurses, develop scientific knowledge (**knowing**), skills (knowing how to **do), an** ethical and relational component (**knowing how to be)** and scientific curiosity (**knowing how to learn**).[27]

Considering these results, it can be highlighted that in terms of **knowledge,** the majority of professionals reported **knowing how to** assess neoplastic wounds, thus emphasizing that they use knowledge based on scientific principles in their care practice.

When it comes to people with neoplastic wounds, an assessment of the patient and the wound is *a sine qua non* for effective care, as without these indicators it is impossible to develop a care plan based on the physical dimensions of the patient's condition. Due to the complexity of these wounds, the initial assessment and recording of the information obtained serve as a subsidy for future assessments, in order to obtain comparisons, so as to help health professionals modify or adjust their interventions, which may be unsuccessful. For this reason, the assessment of neoplastic wounds should be carried out and documented on a daily basis and should include an assessment of all the items listed in Table 1.[5,7,23,28-30]

In addition to the physical aspects, the assessment and recording should include the impact of the wound on the patient's psychological and social well-being and the level of knowledge of the patient and caregiver regarding the care of this injury.[5,7,23,28-30]

It should be emphasized that during the evaluation process, it is necessary to describe the reasons why the interventions were not carried out; conditions that require re-evaluation of the injury, i.e. worsening of the patient's clinical, psychological and social conditions; inability of the caregiver to perform the dressing and reasons why it is impossible to obtain the necessary coverage and products to treat the injury. [5,7,23,28,29-30]

With regard to the items mentioned by the nurses as '**partly known**', i.e. staging, areas of involvement and necessary/appropriate coverings for the lesions, it is believed that the partial knowledge of these aspects may probably be related to the incipience of the subject in question in formal university education, the scarcity of *lato sensu* postgraduate courses in dermatology, oncology and/or palliative care, the lack of national studies on the subject of the study and the weakness of continuing education at the institution *where the* research was carried out.

With regard to the **doing** section, the nurses replied that they did **not** carry out this procedure. This shows an inconsistency with the previous section on **knowledge, since** most of the professionals reported **knowing how to assess** the patient and the neoplastic wound.

In this context, achieving the skills needed to develop autonomous actions has always been a challenge for nursing. However, nurses must have the knowledge and skills to contribute to the quality of care provided to their patients. It is believed that this challenge can be overcome when nurses begin to effectively use the Nursing Process, since it favors the development of specific nursing roles and demonstrates the complexity of care.[31]

In this context, there is the assessment of the patient and the neoplastic lesion, in particular, the patient with cancer who has this type of lesion, which is the subject of this research study. It is through the assessment of the patient and the neoplastic lesion that nurses can detect problems such as: the most frequent skin alteration, the characteristics of the lesion, the most frequent signs and symptoms, the level of knowledge of patients and caregivers about the disease; the difficulties encountered by patients and caregivers in applying a dressing, the psychological, social and spiritual implications of the wound that the patient has, among others.

However, the majority of nurses responded that they did not carry out an assessment of the patient and the neoplastic wound. This leads us to think about some factors that may be considered limiting for this professional practice, namely: problems in staffing, weaknesses in the knowledge obtained in academic training, inability to carry out care with neoplastic wounds, lack of supplies to help in the assessment of the wound, lack of an institutional protocol for the care of neoplastic wounds, or simply the discomfort in carrying out any kind of procedures that are directly related to wounds.

A study of 32 women with vegetating breast wounds found that the criteria used to assess the lesion and clinical symptoms were: wound measurement (height and width); tissue coloration (necrosis = black; fibrin = yellow; granulation = red; epithelialization = pink); digital photography (with a standardized procedure: no *flash*, perpendicular to the wound, average distance of 50 cm to 1m); peripheral skin condition; infectious processes were also used.

pain related to the lesion was assessed using a Visual Analog Scale (VAS) of pain consisting of five items (no pain, mild, moderate, intense and unbearable); odor, bleeding and exudate were assessed using a four-level scale (none, mild, moderate and intense); in addition, bleeding was considered spontaneous when it occurred between two dressing changes with local dressing and no traumatic or induced event when it occurred during the dressing change. The degree to which each symptom was controlled was also scored (controlled, partly controlled and not controlled). Control of the symptoms did not mean that they were treated and cured, but that the discomfort was alleviated by the coverings, local care and treatments.[32]

It is important to emphasize the importance of training as an incentive for the teaching-learning process of nurses in relation to the nursing process for patients with advanced oncological disease. However, it is important to consider the length of training as well as previous accumulated knowledge, since some participants mentioned training and professional experience of one year. Training as a catalyst for the process of learning knowledge has been useful, because through courses, lectures and scientific events, nurses get closer to the methods of assessing and treating wounds and are more likely to apply them in practice.

Table 2 - Frequency distribution of nurses' responses about **knowing** and **doing** basic care for neoplastic wounds. Campina Grande - PB, 2016

Basic care of the neoplastic wound		
	How much do you know	**How much do you make**

	I don't know		I partly know		I know		Yes		No	
	F	%	F	%	F	%	F	%	F	%
l.Calgar sterile gloves for proceed with dressing the wound bed	1	5	1	5	**20**	**90**	**17**	**77**	5	23
2. remove gauze adhered to the wound bed with abundant irrigation using saline solution	1	4	3	14	**18**	**82**	**13**	**59**	9	41
3. irrigate the wound bed with saline solution using a 20 mL syringe/ 40 x 12 cm needle.	2	9	9	41	**11**	**50**	**11**	**50**	**11**	**50**
4. cleaning the wound for superficial removal of bacteria and *debris*	2	9	7	32	**13**	**59**	**12**	**55**	10	45
5. use aseptic technique	1	5	4	18	**17**	77	**14**	**64**	8	36
6. use absorbent dressings	3	14	6	27	**13**	**59**	**13**	**59**	9	41
7. keeping the wound bed moist	3	14	4	18	**15**	**68**	**14**	**64**	8	36
8. remove the spagomortis (fill it with a bandage)	2	9	4	18	**16**	73	**14**	**64**	8	36
90.Promoting symmetrical dressings according to the patient's appearance	3	14	7	32	**21**	**54**	**14**	**64**	8	36

10. protect the dressing with a plastic bag during the spray bath and open it to change only at the bedside (avoiding the dispersion of exudate and microorganisms in the environment).	4	18	**10**	**46**	7	34	9	41	**13**	**59**
TOTAL	22	100	22	100	22	100	22	100	22	100

SOURCE: Research data, 2016

In Table 2, in relation to the segmentation of **knowledge,** the interviewees stated that they knew how to manage cancer wounds in relation to the following items: putting on sterile gloves to proceed with the dressing, removing previous gauze with abundant irrigation using saline solution, irrigating the wound bed with saline solution in a jet using a 20 mL syringe/ 40 x 12 cm needle, cleaning the wound to remove bacteria and *debris from the* surface, use aseptic technique (clean from the least contaminated to the most contaminated), contain/absorb exudate, keep the wound bed moist, eliminate dead space (fill it with dressing) and make dressings symmetrical with the patient's appearance; in one item, the respondents reported that they **knew how to assess, in part**: protecting the dressing with a plastic bag during the sprinkler bath and opening it to change it only at the bedside (avoiding the dispersion of exudate and micro-organisms in the environment).

In terms of how to **do things**, the majority of nurses answered that they carried **out** basic care in relation to the management of cancer lesions in the following items: put on sterile gloves to proceed with the dressing, remove previous gauze with abundant irrigation using saline solution, clean the wound for superficial removal of bacteria and *debris,* use aseptic technique (proceed with cleaning from the least contaminated to the most contaminated environment), contain/absorb exudate, keep the wound bed moist, eliminate dead space (fill it with dressing) and promote dressings that are symmetrical with the patient's appearance and thirteen mentioned that they did **not provide** basic care for neoplastic wounds in the item: protecting the dressing with a plastic bag during the sprinkler bath and opening it to change it only in bed (avoiding the dispersion of exudate and micro-organisms in the environment).

In this section, it is worth noting that in the item "irrigate the wound bed with saline solution in a jet using a 20 mL syringe/ 40 x 12 cm needle", the result was equal, which determines an ambiguity in relation to frequency.

Considering the results highlighted in Table 2, it was observed that the majority of nurses, equally for the **knowing** and **doing** segao, answered that they **knew and did** the basic care for the person with a neoplastic wound.

In chronic wounds, the healing process is long and time-consuming or often non-existent, as these lesions have several factors that hinder healing, such as excess exudate and infectious processes, which tend to recur frequently.[33]

Among the criteria for defining the ideal cover to be used are: providing adequate moisture to the wound bed; protecting the wound against aggression from the outside environment, removing excess exudation to prevent maceration, promoting adequate temperature in the wound bed and being easy to use, apply and manage.[33]

According to the Brazilian Society of Wound and Aesthetic Nursing (SOBENFE)[34] , some basic principles for performing a dressing are: using sterile gloves to proceed with the dressing, cleaning the wound with saline solution using a 20 mL syringe and a 40 x 12 needle to promote irrigation, using coverings that keep the wound bed moist and filling in cavities, tunnels and dead spaces.

The biggest criticism of the moist environment is that there is no information on what constitutes the correct amount of moisture on the surface of wounds, which can produce widely varying amounts of exudate. An intense amount of exudate can promote a culture medium and the growth of microorganisms, cause maceration of the adjacent skin, irritative dermatitis and loss of adherence of the dressing, as well as leaving the patient distressed. Thus, moisture balance in the presence of intense exudate can be achieved by means of absorbent covers, reservoir systems, compressive methods and vacuum therapy.[33]

As well as taking care to absorb the exudate caused by the neoplastic lesion, another basic precaution is to fill in the dead spaces, tunnels and fistulas that develop in the bed or in the peripheral region. These openings are responsible for the formation of sero-hematomas, which can become a medium for culture and the growth of microorganisms, with the consequent infectious process.[35]

A study of 32 women with vegetating breast wounds found that wound care followed wound care protocols adapted to each patient, depending on the characteristics of the wound and the signs and symptoms arising from the wound. The wounds were cleaned with drinking water, saline solution and antiseptic solutions and a variety of primary dressings were used for treatment, including non-adherent and absorbable dressings, secondary dressings and microbial agents.[32]

In addition to the biological factors involved, patients with neoplastic wounds generally experience a sense of mutilation, self-rejection, loss of autonomy and self-esteem, fear, self-care *deficits and* loss of hope in life. In this way, the presence of an oncological lesion can be a determining factor in discrimination, stigma and social rejection. Depending on the characteristics of the wound, the patient tends to shy away from other people so as not to hear unpleasant comments or cause feelings of pity, fear, disgust or displeasure, resulting in a loss of trust, which can have an impact on their quality of life.[36]

A qualitative study of women with breast tumor lesions found that they described some of the challenges they faced living with the neoplastic wound, including: a change in body image, both physical and psychological; clinical management of excessive exudate, foul odor, pain, bleeding and itching; self-loathing and, consequently, a significant impact on mental health and well-being.[37]

In this sense, dressings should be made in such a way that the size and shape are proportionate to the injury, in order to avoid the wound becoming too apparent and affecting the patient's self-image.[38] In view of this, a symmetrical, comfortable, functional and aesthetically acceptable dressing can facilitate the patient's social activity.[36]

Table 3 - Frequency distribution of nurses' responses about **knowing** and **doing** about specific pain control care for neoplastic wounds. Campina Grande - PB, 2016

Specific care you take with the neoplastic wound to control pain

	How much do you know						How much do you make			
	I don't know		I partly know		I know		Yes		No	
	F	%	F	%	F	%	F	%	F	%
1. monitoring the level of pain using the Visual Analog Scale	4	18	3	14	**15**	**68**	**11**	**50**	**11**	**50**
2. consider the use of ice and analgesic medication as prescribed by the doctor	5	23	7	32	**10**	**45**	7	32	**15**	**68**
3. start dressing after 30 minutes for oral analgesia, 5 minutes for subcutaneous or intravenous analgesia, and immediately for topical analgesia as prescribed by the doctor	6	27	6	27	**10**	**46**	5	23	**17**	**77**
4.Carefully remove the adhesives	2	9	3	14	**17**	**77**	**16**	**73**	6	27
5. adjusting the dressing change schedule after the patient has been medicated	5	23	6	27	**11**	**50**	9	41	**13**	**59**
6. assess the need for topical analgesia with 2% lidocaine gel according to medical prescription	7	32	7	32	**8**	**36**	6	27	**16**	**73**
7. not rubbing the wound bed	4	18	4	18	**14**	**64**	**12**	**55**	10	45

8. irrigate the wound bed with saline solution	2	9	3	14	**17**	**77**	**15**	**68**	7	32
9. apply oxide ointment zinc on the edges and around the wound	8	36	6	27	**8**	**37**	5	23	**17**	**77**
10.Observe the need for analgesia after dressing	4	18	7	32	**11**	**50**	8	36	**14**	**64**
11. reassess the need to change the prescribed analgesic regimen	4	18	7	32	**11**	**50**	7	32	**15**	**68**
12. consider, together with the medical team, the need for anti-inflammatory drugs, radiotherapy antiallergic or surgery	7	32	6	27	**9**	**41**	7	32	**15**	**68**
13. record pain assessment using the Visual Analog Scale and analgesia before and after dressing	5	23	7	32	**10**	**45**	6	27	**16**	**73**
14. report to the medical team any cases of pain beyond the control of the recommended approach	5	23	6	27	**11**	**50**	8	36	**14**	**64**
TOTAL	22	100	22	100	22	100	22	100	22	100

SOURCE: Research data, 2016

In Table 3, in relation to the **knowledge** section, the interviewees said they knew all the specific care related to pain control in neoplastic wounds. In this section, it is worth noting that "assess the need for topical analgesia with 2% lidocaine gel", the result was equal between **not knowing** and **not knowing part, giving rise to** ambiguous data in relation to frequency.

In terms of what they **did**, the majority of nurses said that they **did not carry**

out specific care related to pain control in neoplastic wounds: monitoring the level of pain using the Visual Analog Scale; considering the use of ice and analgesic medication according to medical instructions; starting the dressing after 30 minutes for oral analgesia, five minutes for subcutaneous or intravenous analgesia and immediately for topical analgesia; adjusting the dressing change schedule after the patient has already been medicated; applying zinc oxide ointment to the edges and around the wound; observe the need for analgesia after dressing; consider the need, together with the medical team, for anti-inflammatory drugs, anti-algesic radiotherapy or surgery; record the assessment of pain using the Visual Analog Scale and analgesia before and after dressing, and inform the medical team of cases of pain that are beyond the control of the recommended conduct. In this section, it is worth noting that in the item, "monitor the level of pain using the Visual Analog Scale", the result was equal, giving rise to dubious data in relation to frequency.

Considering the results of Table 3, it was observed that **all** the nurses were aware of the specific care applied to pain control for patients with neoplastic wounds; however, the majority replied that they did not apply this knowledge in their care practice.

The goals of pain control include a greater sense of comfort and improved ability to perform daily activities. This requires a comprehensive approach, since pain has multiple factors and requires pharmacological interventions. Therefore, episodes of pain should be promptly re-evaluated, with dose adjustment and investigation into other adjacent causes. Persistent pain related to a neoplastic wound requires ongoing assessment and treatment with regularly administered analgesics.[39]

In this context, as nurses spend more time close to the patient, they are one of the professionals best placed to assess and control pain, in order to promote pain relief and thus contribute to improving the patient's quality of life. It is therefore necessary to use instruments to assess the intensity of pain, taking into account aspects such as physical and cognitive condition, age and the client's way of communicating.[40]

Pain assessment should include intensity, physical characteristics, rhythm and triggering, worsening and relieving factors. In order to understand the condition, it is also essential to know its location, scope, response to current and previous treatments, impact on the performance of daily activities and negative effect on sleep and movement.39

It is worth mentioning that since 2001, the Ministry of Health[39] has recommended palliative measures for pain control, which had already been recommended since 1986 by the World Health Organization, which created the Analgesic Pain Ladder, whose objective is to guide the sequential use of drugs, the gold standard in the treatment of cancer pain and, consequently, in the management of pain in patients with malignant neoplastic wounds.[41-42]

When it comes to pain control in the care of neoplastic wounds, non-pharmacological methods are useful and complement pharmacological therapy; these include wound cleaning techniques, specific dressings and complementary therapies. Among the recommended non-pharmacological methods are: moisten the dressings that are in direct contact with the wound abundantly with saline solution before removing them; use cold saline solution or ice to reduce painful sensations; remove the dressings carefully; irrigate the wound bed with saline solution using a 20 mL syringe with a 40 cm x 12 cm needle; do not rub the wound bed; use non-adherent coverings such as silicone and those that facilitate moisturizing the wound[14-15] , as well as preserving the perilesional skin with a protective barrier using zinc oxide-based ointment as a prophylactic measure in relation to secretion leakage and trauma related to daily dressing changes.[5,29,43]

A study of 32 women with vegetating breast wounds found that a number of measures were taken to reduce pain, including: systemic analgesics for mild pain, weak opioids for moderate pain and strong opioids for severe pain. If pain was expected at the time of dressing changes, Entonox (50% nitrous oxide and 50% oxygen) and a topical anesthetic (EMLA or Xylocaine) were administered. Other treatments such as macerated morphine tablets applied directly to the wound bed and general anesthesia were also carried out.[32]

In view of the context presented by the nurses taking part in the survey, it is believed that ineffective pain control may be related to various causes, among them:

inadequate or non-existent pain assessment due to the accumulation of administrative activities in the face of the care practice that nursing requires; insufficient medical prescription of analgesia; incipient knowledge about systematic pain assessment methods and inability to use specific products and coverings used to reduce pain.

Table 4 - Frequency distribution of nurses' responses about **knowing** and **doing** specific care to control exudate in neoplastic wounds. Campiña Grande - PB, 2016.

Specific care you take with the neoplastic wound to control exudate										
	How much do you know						**How much do you make**			
	I don't know		**I partly know**		**I know**		**Yes**		**No**	
	F	**%**	**F**	**%**	**F**	**%**	**F**	**%**	**F**	**%**
1. collecting material for culture (aspirate and *swab*)	**7**	**32**	**9**	**41**	**6**	**27**	**1**	**5**	**21**	**95**
2. using coal activated/calcium alginate as primary cover and compresses/gauze as secondary cover	6	27	**12**	**54**	4	18	2	9	**20**	**91**
3. use zinc oxide on the edges of the peripheral skin	**11**	**50**	7	32	4	18	2	9	**20**	**91**
TOTAL	22	100	22	100	22	100	22	100	22	100

SOURCE: Research data, 2016.

In Table 4, with regard to the segment of **knowledge,** it can be seen that the majority of nurses answered that they **knew part of the** specific care for controlling exudate in neoplastic wounds in the items: collect material for culture (aspirate or *swab*), use activated charcoal/calcium alginate and compresses/gauze as a secondary covering; on the other hand, in the item "use zinc oxide on macerated skin and wound edges before using antiseptics", the nurses indicated that they **did not know how to** carry out this care.

With regard to the safety of **doing,** all the subjects answered that they did **not**

take specific care to control exudate in the neoplastic wound.

According to the results in Table 4, it can once again be seen that the nurses in the survey have constant weaknesses when it comes to their knowledge and practice of caring for patients with neoplastic wounds. This is worrying because neoplastic wounds have excessive amounts of exudate and, when difficult to control, trigger various complications, including bad odor and myiasis infestation.[16]

Neoplastic wounds generally have large amounts of exudate and when this is not effectively controlled, it can serve as a culture medium for the proliferation of micro-organisms, which contributes to the development of malodors; maceration of the peripheral skin, which in turn contributes to the extension of the lesion; in addition, excessive amounts of exudate can go beyond the primary and secondary coverings, soiling the patient's clothes and causing significant psychosocial problems for the patient. Controlling this symptom reduces odor, avoids soiling the patient's clothes and bedding and provides comfort and confidence for the patient, so it becomes urgent.[16]

The characteristic of the exudate present in wounds is an important indicator that helps in the clinical diagnosis of infection and the choice of topical therapies to be used. To this end, a number of methods are used to assess the exudate present in wounds, which help to quantify and classify the type of exudate in the wound: *Bates - Jensen* Scale and TELER System.33 The gold standard method for analyzing the microbial load is the quantitative culture of viable wound tissue by means of a biopsy and/or *swab* collection carried out using the Levine method, which verifies quantitative cultures.[44]

The type of dressing to be chosen depends on the specifics of the dressing, which vary according to location, size, staging, tissue characteristics and the nature of the injury. Neoplastic wounds are exudative lesions, so absorbent dressings should be used, as they are usually moldable, such as silver foam, hydropolymers, activated charcoal and alginate.[5] As a secondary covering, double gauze or sterile open gauze or surgical compresses associated with a bandage or some type of impermeable covering, such as polyurethane film, are commonly used to occlude and fix the primary covering.[45]

The peripheral skin is that which is circumscribed around the wound, with an extent that varies according to the etiology, location, type, characteristics and magnitude of the wound. Most of the time, this skin is exposed to the action of fluids and exudates from the wound itself and can be cold, dry, thin, scaly, hyperpigmented, macerated and with dermatitis. The edges of the wound, likewise, suffer these repercussions and can appear regular or irregular, adhered or not, thick or thick, friable or with a fibrotic scar. For these reasons, the perilesional skin deserves the same care as the wound bed, according to its specific characteristics.[35] In this sense, authors[9,29,38] emphasize the importance of using zinc oxide-based ointment as a prophylaxis in relation to the toxicity of exudate in the peripheral region, the edges of the lesion and intact skin.

A study of 32 women with neoplastic breast wounds found that microbiological samples were obtained using a curette in each evaluation, in order to identify and quantify aerobic and anaerobic bacteria and characterize the presence of biofilm under fluorescence staining. Exudate was controlled using alginate, hydrofiber and/or hydrocellular as primary covers and surgical pads as secondary covers.[32]

It is worth noting that highly absorbent dressings provide greater comfort and safety for patients with neoplastic wounds, since fluid leakage has an impact on their emotional well-being if it is seen in public, causing them embarrassment.[37]

Thus, it can again be seen that the nurses in this study have a gap in their knowledge about assessment techniques, products and coverings used in the care of patients with neoplastic wounds, which contributes to poor health care.

Table 5 - Frequency distribution of nurses' responses about **knowing** and **doing** specific odor control care for neoplastic wounds. Campina Grande - PB, 2016

Specific care you take with the neoplastic wound to control odor					
	How much do you know			**How much you make**	
	I don't know	**I partly know**	**I know**	**Yes**	**No**

1.Clean with saline solution and antiseptic with chlorohexidine	F	%	F	%	F	%	F	%	F	%
	1	5	6	27	**15**	**68**	**18**	**82**	4	18
2. remove antiseptic with a jet of saline solution and then keep gauze soaked in aluminum hydroxide on the wound bed	6	27	**9**	**41**	7	32	4	18	**18**	**82**
3. use silver sulfadizine on the lesion bed and then occlude with gauze soaked in liquid petroleum jelly	**11**	**5**	6	27	5	23	3	14	**19**	**86**
4.Apply activated charcoal to the lesion bed and cover with gauze moistened with saline solution.	**10**	**46**	6	27	5	23	2	9	**20**	**91**
5. apply 0.8% metronidazole gel according to medical prescription, for grade I odor, to the wound bed and then cover with gauze soaked in Vaseline	7	32	3	14	**12**	**55**	**11**	**50**	**11**	**50**
6. if necessary, perform a scarotomy on necrotic tissue and apply metronidazole gel, as prescribed by the doctor, for grade II odor	**10**	**46**	11	50	1	5	1	5	**21**	**95**
7. consider with the medical team, the possibility of associating systemic metronidazole (intravenous or oral) with topical use, for grade III odor	**12**	**55**	6	27	4	18	2	9	**20**	**91**
TOTAL	22	100	22	100	22	100	22	100	22	100

SOURCE: Research data, 2016

In Table 5, with regard to the **knowledge** section, it can be seen that the majority of nurses stated that they **did not know** the specific care regarding odor in neoplastic wounds in the items: use silver sulphadizine in gauze and occlude with gauze soaked in liquid vaseline, use activated charcoal in gauze moistened with 0.9% SF if necessary, perform a *square* technique (escharotomy) on necrotic tissue and apply metronidazole gel as directed by the doctor and consider, together with the medical team, the possibility of combining systemic metronidazole (intravenous or oral) with topical use. With regard to the item 'remove antiseptic with a jet of 0.9% saline solution and keep gauze soaked in aluminum hydroxide on the wound bed', most of the nurses answered that they **knew.**

With regard to the **doing** section, most of the subjects answered that they **did not take** specific care of the odor of the neoplastic wound in the following items: remove antiseptic with a jet of 0.9% saline and keep gauze soaked in aluminum hydroxide in the wound bed, use silver sulfadizine in gauze and occlude with gauze soaked in liquid petroleum jelly, use activated charcoal in gauze moistened with 0.9% saline, if necessary, perform a *square* technique (escharotomy) on necrotic tissue and apply metronidazole gel as prescribed by the doctor and consider, together with the medical team, the possibility of combining systemic metronidazole (intravenous or oral) with topical use.

In this same section, it is worth noting that in the item "apply 0.8% metronidazole gel as prescribed by the doctor on gauze soaked in Vaseline and apply to the wound bed" the result was the same for the study, leading to an ambiguity regarding the frequency.

It is possible to see a repetition of the results in the **knowing** and **doing** sections of this study, since the majority of nurses are unaware of the measures used to control the symptoms of neoplastic wounds, particularly odor, as highlighted in the table above. This leads us to believe, once again, that there is a gap in health education.

The foul odor is considered by patients to be the most distressing symptom, as it can lead to embarrassment, feelings of disgust, depression, social isolation, have a detrimental effect on sexual expression and cause problems in relationships. Odor is detected by olfactory receptors located in the nasal region and is processed both consciously and subconsciously, triggering vomiting reflexes. On a subconscious level, the foul odor affects the experience of taste and aroma. This obviously has a profoundly negative impact on the patient, decreasing their appetite and enjoyment of food, which contributes to marked weight loss.[6-7,14]

Odor is a symptom that is very difficult to assess. In this sense, authors[5] have described a clinical indicator for quantifying odor, which is used in conjunction with a patient-focused indicator, the aim of which is to determine the impact of odor on the patient. In this way, the indicator has become an important assessment tool and for this reason, the National Cancer Institute[5] , based on the TELER system, has constructed an odor assessment scale for neoplastic wounds, which classifies odor into three levels, namely Grade I, II and III.

To treat the odor, the first step is to clean the lesion with an antiseptic such as chlorhexidine, which belongs to the biguanide group and acts on gram-positive and gram-negative microorganisms.[35] Silver sulfadiazine 1% and metronidazole in various presentations can be used as primary coverings.

According to the *European Pressure Ulcer Advisory Panel and the National Pressure Ulcer Advisory Panel*[44] , some recommendations should be valued by health professionals in the control of wound infections, namely: consider the use of topical antiseptics in conjunction with maintenance debridement in order to control and eradicate the biofilm that is suspected to be present in difficult-to-heal wounds; consider the use of topical antiseptics in wounds that are not expected to heal and are highly colonized/infected topically and consider the use of silver sulfadiazine in highly contaminated or infected wounds until definitive debridement is performed. In addition to these pharmacological modalities, patients also benefit from the use of compresses soaked in aluminum hydroxide.

If the patient has a wound with necrotic tissue with a hardened, inelastic appearance and a circular constricting crust, which compromises capillary refill and blood supply, impairing tissue oxygenation, the professional can make vertical and horizontal relaxing incisions on the wound (escharotomy). In addition to improving blood perfusion, escharotomy in necrotic wounds facilitates the penetration of products into the wound, which contributes to absortion.[46]

A study of 32 women with vegetating breast wounds found that a number of measures had been taken to reduce odor, including: cleaning the wound with polyhexanidamethyl biguanide (PHMB)-based solutions; primary coatings such as activated charcoal, silver impregnations, hydrocellulose containing silver nanocrystals and topical antimicrobials such as metronidazole.[32]

Odor is a serious problem that affects both the body image and the quality of life of patients with neoplastic wounds, as well as those around them. For this reason, nurses need to be properly trained and prepared to control this symptom and to intervene in the emotional demands that the patient may present.

Table 6 - Frequency distribution of nurses' responses about **knowing** and **doing** specific care to control bleeding in neoplastic wounds. Campiña Grande - PB, 2016

Specific care you take with the neoplastic wound to control bleeding										
	How much do you know						**How much do you make**			
	I don't know		**I partly know**		**I know**		**Yes**		**No**	
	F	**%**	**F**	**%**	**F**	**%**	**F**	**%**	**F**	**%**
1.Apply pressure directly over the bleeding vessels with gauze, compresses or towels	2	9	4	18	**16**	**73**	**16**	**73**	6	27
2. consider applying cold saline solution	2	9	7	32	**13**	**59**	**13**	**59**	9	41

3. consider a hemostatic dressing based on porcine gelatin (Gelfoam)	**13**	**59**	5	23	4	18	1	5	**21**	**95**
4.Consider calcium alginate	9	41	**10**	**45**	3	14	2	9	**20**	**91**
5. consider applying adrenaline (injectable solution) topically to bleeding points as prescribed by the doctor	6	27	**9**	**41**	7	32	5	23	**17**	**77**
6. keeping the environment moist, avoiding adherence of gauze to the wound bed	3	14	4	18	**15**	**68**	**12**	**55**	10	45
7. check with the medical team the possibility of treatment with a systemic coagulant such as aminocaproic acid	**11**	**50**	8	36	3	14	2	9	**20**	**91**
8. check with the medical team the possibility of treatment with surgical intervention	6	27	**10**	**46**	6	27	5	23	**17**	**77**
9. check with the medical team the possibility of treatment with anti-hemorrhagic radiotherapy	8	36	**11**	**50**	3	14	4	18	**18**	**82**
10. check with the medical team the possibility of palliative sedation treatment for cases of intense bleeding accompanied by agitation, despair and distress on the part of the patient	7	32	**9**	**41**	6	27	4	18	**18**	**82**

TOTAL	22	100	22	100	22	100	22	100	22	100

SOURCE: Research data, 2016

In Table 6, with regard to the **knowledge** section, it can be seen that the majority of nurses answered that they **partly knew about** specific care in relation to bleeding from neoplastic wounds in the following items: consider calcium alginate, consider adrenaline (injectable solution) topically on the bleeding points according to medical prescription, check with the medical team the possibility of treatment with surgical intervention, check with the medical team the possibility of treatment with anti-hemorrhagic radiotherapy and check, with the medical team, the possibility of treatment with palliative sedation for cases of intense bleeding accompanied by agitation, despair and anguish on the part of the patient and the majority said they **did not know how to** consider a hemostatic dressing based on porcine gelatin (Gelfoam) to control bleeding.

With regard to the **doing** section, most of the subjects answered that they did **not take** specific care of the bleeding in the neoplastic wound.

According to the results shown in Table 6, we can once again see that the research subjects had insufficient knowledge about controlling the symptoms of neoplastic wounds, now involving the management of bleeding. This is something that deserves a lot of attention, since bleeding can cause the patient to feel anxious, restless and distressed, especially those who are phobic; but above all, it can cause severe hemodynamic changes, leading to death.

Tumor hemorrhages are generally the most intense forms of bleeding and the most difficult to manage, which is why the precise location of the bleeding site, combined with the definition of the tumor's staging, is essential in order to take the most appropriate course of action.[47]

In these circumstances, the use of non-adherent dressings, such as silicone dressings, is recommended as a priority to prevent bleeding, as they avoid adherence to the wound bed and possible bleeding during dressing changes. Non-adherent dressings are applied directly to the bed of the lesion and do not cause significant trauma at the time of removal, although they do require secondary coverage. Other important factors that should be emphasized to prevent bleeding are irrigation with saline solution of the previous dressing (when adherent dressings are used) and cleaning the wound with irrigation technique.[7,14,23,26,48-50]

To control bleeding, a variety of hemostatic agents can be applied topically or systemically to control bleeding. These hemostatic agents vary according to their application and mechanisms. Examples include natural hemostatics (calcium alginates, collagen and oxidized cellulose), coagulants (absorbable gelatin sponge powder or topical thrombin), sclerosing agents (silver nitrate, trichloroacetic acid), vasoconstrictors (epinephrine), inhibitors (tranexamic acid, fibrinolytics) and astringents (alum solution and sucralfate).[7]

Other pharmacological modalities that can be used by the team are aminocaproic acid and tranexamic acid, which act systematically; while sutures, pinches and cauterizations are local hemostatic surgical interventions, generally used when there is a rupture of important vessels.[7,14,26,51-55]

Palliative radiotherapy aims to treat the primary tumor or metastases locally, without influencing the patient's survival, and is mainly used to control pain and bleeding. Indications for anti-hemorrhagic radiotherapy include control of oral bleeding, epistaxis, metrorrhagia, hematuria, vaginal and rectal bleeding; it is also used to control the rapid growth of exophytic tumors.[56-58]

A study of 32 women with vegetating breast wounds found that some measures were taken to reduce bleeding, including: removing the dressing gently, using non-stick dressings (silicone), alginate as a hemostatic dressing and adrenaline as a local and systemic vasoconstrictor.[32]

Massive bleeding is very painful for the patient and their family, not only because of the hemorrhage, but above all because profuse blood loss can cause the patient's imminent death. In this sense, a strategic plan should be developed together with the patient and family when such an event is considered a possibility. After a careful assessment of the patient's circumstances, the plan should include: explanation of the possibility of profuse bleeding to caregivers and family members; guidance on the attitudes that should be taken by the family at the time of bleeding; leaving dark-colored towels and a basin near the patient's bedside; preparation of an emergency *kit,* including sedative drugs; access to the emergency transport service and open lines of communication with appropriate specialized centers where the emergency can be quickly called.[16]

Table 7 - Frequency distribution of nurses' responses about **knowing** and **doing** specific care to control necrosis of neoplastic wounds. Campiña Grande - PB, 2016

Specific care you take with the neoplastic wound to control necrosis										
	How much do you know						**How much do you make**			
	I don't know		**I partly know**		**I know**		**Yes**		**No**	
	F	**%**	**F**	**%**	**F**	**%**	**F**	**%**	**F**	**%**
1. assess the need for debridement, according to the patient's ability.	3	14	**11**	50	8	36	6	27	**16**	73
2. choosing the form of debridement (mechanical, chemical, autolytic)	3	14	**12**	55	7	54	7	32	**15**	68
TOTAL	22	100	22	100	22	100	22	100	22	100

SOURCE: Research data, 2016

In Table 7, with regard to the **knowing** section, it can be seen that the majority of nurses answered that they **knew part of the** specific care related to the control of necrosis in neoplastic wounds in the following items: assessing debridement needs, according to the patient's capacity and choosing the form of debridement (mechanical, chemical, autolytic). In the **doing** section, the majority of subjects answered that they did **not take** specific care to control necrosis in neoplastic wounds.

According to the results mentioned in Table 7, it can once again be seen that the research subjects had insufficient knowledge about controlling the symptoms of neoplastic wounds, now involving the management of necrosis.

When it comes to caring for necrosis, the best course of action is autolytic and enzymatic debridement[59] , but the risks and benefits of this procedure for patients with malignant neoplastic wounds must be assessed, since the friability of the lesions can lead to a potential risk of massive bleeding.[51,59]

In this sense, some factors must be taken into account before debridement is carried out, such as: the area to be debrided, the presence of local infections, the vascularization and neovascularization of the site, the risks of bleeding during or after the procedure, odor control resistant to previous therapies and the patient's general condition.[51]

According to the Ministry of Health[5] , nurses should assess the need for debridement considering the patient's functional capacity, as well as selecting the method: autolytic, enzymatic, mechanical or surgical. If necessary, authors point out[60] , that the debridement of malignant neoplastic wounds should be carried out in the operating room, given the need to use hemostatic equipment, such as electrocautery, unless the patient is on anticoagulants and/or is undergoing chemotherapy and/or radiotherapy; in these circumstances, the doctor is the one who carries out this procedure.

In these wounds, the *debris* can be removed by maintaining a moist environment, by gently cleaning the necrotic areas or by using jets of saline solution at a pressure of 8 to 15 *psi (pound force per square inch)*.[60] When the tumor has extensive necrotic tissue, surgical debridement may be indicated in order to prevent infection, control exudate and odor; however, consideration should be given to cases in which the patient is in palliative care, since this procedure generates greater physical and emotional suffering for the patient and the family.

A survey[21] carried out with 20 nurses at the same institution where the study was carried out found that the participants mentioned that the service where they cared for neoplastic wounds did not provide specific materials and/or dressings to control necrosis, leaving the family - only those with favorable financial conditions - responsible for buying such products, which would control this symptom, considered one of the most devastating and the source of various complications. This result points to a fragile and psychosocially limited Brazilian health policy, especially for terminally ill patients.[21]

An intervention study of 12 women with malignant wounds found that autolytic debridement was more beneficial than surgical debridement. The dressings were applied with hydrogel as the primary dressing and foam as the secondary dressing. Nine women (75%), after the intervention period, showed a reduction in the size of the wound and the appearance of granulation tissue and epithelialization; one patient had her wound completely healed and in three patients (25%), the wounds increased in size and showed less vascularization and granulation tissue, as well as more fibrosis, yellow and black necrosis, and infection. This may have been because these three women were no longer receiving antineoplastic treatment.[61]

The healing of malignant tumor wounds in the aforementioned study was observed during the intervention period, a finding not reported in the literature as far as we know. In some studies[7-8,14,23,62] authors state that healing malignant fungal wounds is an unrealistic goal, and that wound care is solely palliative. Therefore, it is important to state that through this intervention, despite being an old publication, researchers have managed to optimize healing, with an increase in vascularization, granulation and epithelialization and a reduction in wound size. In order to update these data, EPUAP and NPUAP[44] recommend that health professionals consider using hydrogel to treat wounds with dry beds.[44]

A study[63] carried out on four patients with cancer verified the efficacy of active *Leptospermum* honey paste (ALH) on malignant lesions. Total healing of the lesions was observed in two patients and in the other two there was a reduction in the intensity of pain and the size of the lesion, eradication of odor, a reduction in liquefaction tissue and an increase in granulation tissue. Despite being an old experience report, EPUAP and NPUAP44 recommend that health professionals consider using honey on highly contaminated or infected wounds until definitive debridement has been carried out.

Table 8 - Distribution of the frequencies of the nurses' responses about **knowing** and **doing about the** specific care performed to control the cutaneous fistula in a neoplastic wound Campina Grande - PB. 2016

Specific care you take with the neoplastic wound to control the cutaneous fistula										
	How much do you know						**How much do you make**			
	I don't know		**I partly know**		**I know**		**Yes**		**No**	
	F	%	F	%	F	%	F	%	F	%
1.Apply zinc oxide to the skin around the fistula	4	18	**12**	55	6	27	3	14	**19**	86
2. adapting, where possible, the use of collection bags in high-drainage fistulas and hydrocolloid sheets around the skin	4	18	**10**	46	8	36	8	36	**14**	64
3. perform absorbent dressing with activated charcoal and/or calcium alginate as primary cover and compress/gauze as secondary cover	4	18	**12**	54	6	28	5	23	**17**	77
TOTAL	22	100	22	100	22	100	22	100	22	100

SOURCE: Research data, 2016

In Table 8, with regard to the **knowledge** section, it can be seen that the majority of nurses answered that they **partly knew about** specific care in relation to the control of cutaneous fistulae in neoplastic wounds in the following items: Apply zinc oxide to the skin around the fistula; adapt, when possible, use of collection bags in high-drainage fistulas, with hydrocolloid sheets around the skin and perform absorptive dressing with activated charcoal and/or calcium alginate as primary coverage and compress/gauze as secondary coverage. And in the **do** section, most of the subjects answered that they did **not take** specific care to control the cutaneous fistula in the neoplastic wound.

Once again, the data points to a fragile, gaping and incipient nursing care practice, which urgently calls for the creation and implementation of continuing education in the service.

Cutaneous fistulae can arise as a result of complications from treatments such as surgery, brachytherapy, radiotherapy, or even disease progression and/or recurrence. In general, the formation of fistulas in malignant tumor wounds is directly related to the progression of the cancer. The main types of cancer that are most likely to form fistulas are head and neck cancer (oro-cutaneous and esophago-cutaneous fistulas) and gynecological cancer (external fistula, so-called cutaneous fistula and internal fistula). The presence of fistulas aggravates the wound, making it more exudative and fetid, as well as causing erosion of the peripheral skin.[64-65]

Nursing care related to the presence of fistulas in malignant tumor wounds primarily involves assessing the path and condition of the fistula, treatment, and educating the patient and their caregiver. One of the most essential precautions is to evaluate the effluent in terms of color, presence of odor and volume drained in 24 hours. According to the volume of exudate, the fistula can be classified as low output (less than 500 mL) and high output (more than 500 mL). Care in the management of fistulas should take into account that, if there is a flow of up to 250 mL/24 hours, it can be contained with gauze and/or highly absorbent dressings; in the case of larger drains, it is recommended to use stoma collectors, including pediatric ones, which are smaller and adapt better to the patient's body. Due to the irregular shape of these wounds, these products can be useful for shaping the edges of the lesion so that the collection bag can be attached to receive the effluent. It is essential to protect the skin around the fistula and this can be done by applying hydrocolloid sheets, sealants, barrier cream and/or paste.

When fistulas have an odor, the use of activated charcoal and/or gelling capsules for colostomies (which disintegrate in the liquid medium and control the odor of the effluent) should be considered.[65] In addition, the nurse and medical team can discuss the possibility of using systemic metronidazole when faced with more offensive odors or other drugs, such as hyoscine and octreotide, which are also recommended in palliative care. People with advanced wounds at risk of developing fistulas are generally malnourished, have hypoalbuminemia (< 20 mg/dL) or negative protein balance, significant anemia (Hb < 8) and use high doses of immunosuppressive drugs.[7] For this reason, considering the entire environment of the person affected by advanced cancer and the presence of a malignant tumor wound, assessing their nutritional status and their hydroelectrolytic balance through laboratory tests is mandatory.[66] **Table 9** - Frequency distribution of nurses' responses about **knowing** and **doing** specific care to control pruritus in neoplastic wounds. Campina Grande - PB, 2016

Specific care you take with the neoplastic wound to control pruritus										
	How much do you know						**How much do you make**			
	I don't know		**I partly know**		**I know**		**Yes**		**No**	
	F	**%**	**F**	**%**	**F**	**%**	**F**	**%**	**F**	**%**
l.Investigate the cause of the itching	3	14	8	36	**11**	**50**	7	32	**15**	68
2. consider using hypoallergenic adhesives (micropore)	0	0	5	23	**17**	77	**16**	73	6	27
3. use dexamethasone cream 0.1% on the itchy areas as prescribed by your doctor	6	27	7	32	**9**	**41**	5	23	**17**	**73**
4. use 1% silver sulphadiazine as prescribed by a doctor for cutaneous candidiasis in areas of hyperemia around the wound associated with whitish patches	7	32	**8**	36	7	32	5	23	**17**	**77**

5. consider reducing the interval between dressings to avoid this symptom	5	23	7	32	**10**	**45**	5	23	**17**	**77**
6. If pruritus persists, consider introducing systemic therapy with the medical team.	6	27	7	32	**9**	**41**	6	27	**16**	**73**
TOTAL	22	100	22	100	22	100	22	100	22	100

SOURCE: Research data, 2016

In Table 9, in relation to the segmentation of **knowledge**, the majority of interviewees stated that they **knew** about the care taken to control pruritus in cancer lesions in relation to the items: Investigate the cause of pruritus, consider the use of hypoallergenic adhesives (micropore), consider reducing the dressing interval to avoid this symptom and if pruritus persists, consider with the medical team the introduction of systemic therapy. On the other hand, in the item 'use silver sulphadiazine 1% as prescribed by the doctor, for cutaneous candidiasis in areas of hyperemia around the wound associated with whitish patches', the respondents indicated that they **partly knew.**

With regard to the action of **doing**, the majority of subjects answered that they did **not carry out** clinical management in relation to pruritus control in the items: Investigate the cause of pruritus, use dexamethasone cream 0.1% in the areas of pruritus as prescribed by the doctor, use silver sulfadiazine 1% as prescribed by the doctor, for cutaneous candidiasis in the areas of hyperemia around the wound associated with whitish patches, consider reducing the interval between dressings to avoid this symptom and if itching persists, consider introducing systemic therapy together with the medical team and eight mentioned that **they** controlled itching in the item consider using hypoallergenic patches (micropore).

The results in Table 9 show that the majority of nurses are **aware of** and **do not** control pruritus. Once again, the data is similar, i.e. it seems that the problems faced by the nurses in this study are poor staffing levels, lack of continuing education in the service, lack of institutional protocols for the care of neoplastic wounds and lack of supplies, materials, products and medicines for the clinical management of these lesions.

Pruritus is related to the release of histamines by the inflammatory process of the wound or to the use of products on the lesion causing an allergic process in the wound bed or in tissues around the wound.[14,26,54,66-67] In this situation, the use of 0.1% dexamethasone cream on the wound bed and peripheral region is recommended in order to minimize manifestations in the event of allergic processes[5] . Other authors[66] also recommend the use of hydrogel to keep the wound bed hydrated and, finally, the use of *Transcutaneous Electrical Nerve Stimulation* (TENS), a non-invasive method that is easy to apply and prevents central hypersensitivity caused by the inflammatory process and activates the release of endogenous opioids, thus reducing itching and pain.

Finally, it is worth mentioning a multicenter study[8] with 700 oncology nurses, which found that these professionals had some difficulties when dealing with people with tumor wounds, namely: uncertainty about the correct use of dressings in relation to the treatment of these lesions; inexperience in caring for this type of wound; lack of evidence-based guidelines and lack of continuing education in primary and hospital care; and lack of specific supplies, materials and products for the treatment of tumor wounds.

Table 10 - Distribution of nurses' responses about **knowing** and **doing about the** records of actions taken with neoplastic wounds. Campina Grande - PB, 2016

Record of the nursing actions you carry out on the patient and the neoplastic wound										
	How much do you know						**How much do you make**			
	I don't know		**I partly know**		**I know**		**Yes**		**No**	
	F	%	F	%	F	%	F	%	F	%
1.Document wound and patient assessment	7	32	7	32	**8**	**36**	7	32	**15**	**68**

2. document all interventions carried out	4	18	1	5	**17**	**77**	**15**	**68**	7	32
3. documenting patient and/or family education, highlighting points of difficulty in understanding and skill	3	14	3	14	**16**	**72**	**16**	**73**	6	27
4. documenting the results obtained	5	23	6	27	**11**	**50**	7	32	**15**	**68**
TOTAL	22	100	22	100	22	100	22	100	22	100

SOURCE: Research data, 2016.

In Table 10, with regard to the **knowledge** section, it can be seen that all the nurses answered that they **knew how to** record the actions taken with the patient and the neoplastic wound in the following items: documenting the assessment of the wound and the patient, documenting all the interventions carried out, documenting the education carried out with the patient and/or family, pointing out any points of difficulty in understanding and skill, and documenting the results obtained.

With regard to the **doing** section, half of the nurses replied that they **didn't** document the assessment of the wound and the patient, nor did they record the results obtained; however, the other half replied that they documented all the interventions carried out and documented the education given to the patient and/or family, signaling points of difficulty in understanding and skill.

According to the results highlighted in Table 10, there is once again an inconsistency between **knowing** and **doing,** given that all the nurses replied that they 'knew' how to document aspects related to the wound and the patient, but some of them mentioned that they **didn't** assess the wound and the patient and didn't document the results obtained.

With this in mind, Resolution No. 429/2012 of the Federal Nursing Council[68] provides for the recording of nursing actions in the patient's medical record, whether traditional or electronic, and states in Article 1 that it is the responsibility and duty of nursing professionals to record in the patient's medical record and in other documents specific to the area, information regarding the care process and the management of the work process, which is necessary to ensure the continuity and quality of care.

A study[69] of 71 medical records found that, in general, there was a lack of information about the characteristics of the wound, such as: type of tissue (65%), type of exudate (85%), measurement of the lesion (100%), aspects related to the wound bed and peripheral skin (80%) and complaints of pain (98%). In addition, most of the nursing prescriptions were not checked (75%) and had illegible writing (54%). It is worth noting that the psychosocial-spiritual dimension was only included in one medical record. Furthermore, in all the medical records (100%), the notes were in abbreviated form, 59% were unclear, 35% had grammatical language errors and 80% did not have correct terminology.[69]

When it comes to wound care, the systematic recording of the assessment of the wound, the patient and the type of dressing used are the cornerstones for controlling the symptoms of neoplastic wounds. These records must be made with criteria and with instruments that make it easier to note the characteristics and factors that interfere with symptom control, so it is essential to standardize the terms. It is therefore understood that the construction and implementation of protocols for the control of symptoms resulting from neoplastic wounds are essential, as well as training for the multi-professional team.69

The nursing register is one of the means of proving the legal exercise of the profession. In this way, incorrect completion and, above all, the lack of periodicity and continuity are factors that make it irreversibly impossible to carry out any kind of evaluation, certification, creation of indicators and even investigations and expert opinions that could even provide legal support for the professional and the institution.69

In view of the above, it is essential that the participating nurses become aware of the importance of recording nursing interventions and adopt attitudes that are in line with the ethical principles of the profession.

FINAL CONSIDERATIONS

In general, the results obtained in this study showed that nurses have gaps in their knowledge of content and techniques for assessing and treating patients with neoplastic wounds. In addition, it was found that nurses do not carry out some of the care that is relevant to this clientele.

The analysis showed that nurses have limited knowledge to assess the specificities of the lesion and the patient, the indication of coverage and the type of dressing to be used to control the signs and symptoms of these lesions. These limitations are probably related to the lack of permanent education in the health service and continuing education in related areas, such as Dermatology, Stomatherapy, Palliative Care and others.

Another worrying aspect is the omission of nursing care for these patients. It is believed that the failure to carry out the assessment and treatment of patients with neoplastic wounds is related to a number of factors, including: a lack of knowledge regarding the contents and techniques of neoplastic wound care; an increase in workload due to management activities; poor planning of the sizing of staff, supplies and materials for wound assessment, as well as scarce products, substances and coverings in the health service.

In this sense, the results of this study point to the need for continuing education in the health service, the *locus of* the research, in order to train the nursing team to monitor patients with neoplastic lesions, as well as the structuring of a palliative care unit, with the necessary human and material resources, the creation and implementation of care protocols that guide the practice of evaluation and therapeutic methods in the care of people with neoplastic wounds, their families and caregivers.

This study has some limitations: the sample was small and only nurses from the same institution were surveyed, but the objectives were met. For this reason, the study needs to be replicated, after refining the instrument, with a larger sample and in other health institutions, in order to gain an overview of how knowledge and practice of caring for patients with neoplastic wounds is being carried out.

Another limitation of the study is related to the discussion of the results, in terms of the scarcity of comparative data with other studies. In this sense, it is worth pointing out that the studies published nationally and internationally on the subject generally have a bibliographic design, which contributes to low levels of evidence, making comparison impossible, which is considered a *sine qua non* condition for confirming or refuting the hypotheses of the research in question.

Although we recognize the limitations of the study, it is essential to take the results as a way of reflecting on the importance of health education in the process of training nurses. To this end, education also needs to be comprehensive and interdisciplinary, based on critical-reflective references, enabling the acquisition of competences and skills that guarantee action geared towards the person with a neoplastic wound in their subjectivity.

REFERENCES

l.Vasconcelos AMN, Gomes MMF. Demographic transition: the Brazilian experience.
Epidemiol Serv Saúde [Internet] 2012. [cited 2016 June 02] 21(4):539-48. DOI:
http://dx.doi.org/10.5123/S1679-49742012000400003

2 Guimarães RM, Muzi CD, Teixeira MP, Pinheiro SS. The transition of cancer mortality in Brazil and strategic decision-making in women's health public policies. *Rev Pol Pub* [Internet] 2016. [cited 2016 June 04] 20(1):33-50.
DOI: http://dx.doi.org/10.18764/2178-2865.v20n1p35-50

3 Marques CLTQ, Barreto CL, Morais VLL, Lima Júnior NF. Oncology: a multidisciplinary approach. Recife: Carpe Diem Ediçoes, 2015.

4. National Cancer Institute. Brazil. Estimate 2016/2017: Incidence of Cancer in Brazil. Rio de Janeiro: INCA, 2016.

5 National Cancer Institute. Brazil. Treatment and control of tumor wounds and pressure ulcers in advanced cancer. Palliative Care Series. Rio de Janeiro: INCA, 2011.

6 Santos CMC, pimenta CAM, Nobre MRC. A systematic review of topical treatments to control the odor of malignant fungating wounds. *J Pain Symptom Manage* [Internet] 2010. [cited 2016 June 11] 39(6):1065-76. DOI: 10.1016/j.jpainsymman.2009.11.31

7 Woo K, Sibbald RG. Local wound care for malignant and palliative wounds. *Adv Skin Wound Care* [Internet] 2010 Sept. [cited 2016 June 15] 23(9):417-28. DOI: 10.1097/01.ASW.0000383206.32244.e2

8 Probst S, Arber A, Faithfull S. Malignant fungating wounds: a survey of nurses' clinical practice in Switzerland. *Eur J Oncol Nurs* [Internet] 2009. [cited 2016 June 19] 13:295-8. DOI: 10.1016/j.ejon.2009.03.008

9 Gozzo TO, Tahan FP, Andrade M, Nascimento TG, Prado MAS. Occurrence and management of neoplastic wounds in women with advanced breast cancer. *Esc Anna Nery* [Internet] 2014 [cited 2016 June 21] 18(2):270-6. DOI:
http://dx.doi.org/10.5935/1414-8145.20140039

10Lisboa IND, Valença MP. Characterization of Patients with Neoplastic Wounds. *Estima* [Internet] 2016 [cited 2016 June 28] 14(1):21-8. DOI: 10.5327/Z1806- 3144201600010004

11Gethin G, Grocott P, Probst S, Clarke E. Current practice in the management of wound odour: an international survey. *Int J Nurs Stud* [Internet] 2013. Jun [cited 2016 July 03] 51(6):865-74. DOI: 10.1016/j.ijnurstu.2013.10.013

12Gibson S, Green J. Review of patients' experiences with fungating wounds and associated quality of life. *J Wound Care* [Internet] 2013. May [cited 2016 July 05] 22(5):265-72. DOI: 10.12968/jowc.2013.22.5.265 17.

13Probst S, Arber A, Faithfull S. Malignant fungating wounds: the meaning of living in an unbounded body. *Eur J Oncol Nurs* [Internet] 2013. Feb [cited 2016 July 10] 17(1):38-45. DOI: 10.1016/j.ejon.2012.02.001

14Alexander S. Malignant fungating wounds: key symptoms and psychosocial. *J Wound Care* [Internet] 2009 Aug [cited 2016 July 13] 18(8):325-9. DOI: 10.12968/jowc.2009.18.8.43631

15Alexander S. Maliganant fungating wounds: managing pain, bleending and psychosocial issues. *J Wound Care* [Internet] 2009 Oct. [cited July 18] 18(10):418- 25. DOI: 10.12968/jowc.2009.18.10.44603

16Alexander S. Malignant fungating wounds: managing malodor and exudate. *J Wound Care* [Internet] 2009 Sept [cited 2016 July 30] 18(9):374-82. DOI: 10.12968/jowc.2009.18.9.44305

17Blakely AM, Mcphillips J, Miner TJ. Surgical palliation for malignant disease requiring locoregional control. *Ann Palliatt Med* [Intenet] 2015 Apr [cited 2016 Aug 06] 4(1):48-53. DOI: 10.3978/j.issn.2224-5820.2015.04.03

18Beh SY, Leow LC. Fungating breast cancer and other malignant wounds: epidemiology, assessment and management. *Expert Rev Qual Life Cancer Care.*
[Internet] 2016. Mar [cited 2016 Aug 10] 1(2):137-44. DOI: org/10.1080/23809000.2016.1162660

19Maida V, Alexander S, Case AA, Fakhraei P. Malignant wound management.
Public Health Emerg [Internet] 2016. Jun [cited 2016 Aug 12] 1:12. DOI: 10.21037/phe.2016.06.15

20Tilley C, Lipson J, Ramos M. Palliative wound care for malignant fungating wounds: holistic considerations at end-of-life. *Nurs Clin N Am* [Internet] 2016 [cited 2016 Aug 17]. 51(3):513-31. Available from: https://www.ncbi.nlm.nih.gov/pubmed/27497023

21Agra G, Santos JP, Sousa ATO, Gouveia BLA, Brito, DTF, Macêdo EL et al. Malignant neoplastic wounds: clinical management performed by nurses. *Int Arch Med* [Internet] 2016 [cited 2017 Feb 12] 9(344):1-13. DOI: http://dx.doi.org/10.3823/2215

22Walsh AF, Bradley MMSN, Cavallito K. Management of fungating tumors and pressure ulcers in a patient with stage iv cutaneous malignant melanoma. *J Hosp Palliat Nurs* [Internet] 2014 June [cited Aug 18]16(4):208-14. DOI: 10.1097/NJH.0000000000000076

23Merz T, Klein C, Uebach B, Kern M, Ostgathe C, Bükki J. Fungating wounds: multidimentional challenge in palliative care. *Breast Care*

[Internet] 2011 Feb. [cited 2016 Aug 20] 6(1):21-4. DOI: 10.1159/000324923

24. Agra G, Medeiros MVS, Brito DTF, Sousa ATO, Formiga NS, Costa MML. Knowledge and practice of nurses in the care of patients with malignant tumor wounds. *Rev Cuid.* [Internet] 2017. Dec. [cited 2017 Dec 30] 8(3):1849-62. DOI http://dx.doi.org/10.15649/cuidarte.v8i3.441

25González RC, Robles CC, Gómez FC, Uría AD, Saíz BF, España MVG et al. Manual de prevención y cuidados locales de heridas crónicas. Central Health Service, 2011. 223p.

26Vaquer LM. Management of cutaneous ulcers of tumor origin; cutánides. *Rev Int Grupos Invest Oncol* [Internet] 2012. Mar [cited 2016 Aug 23] 1(2):52-9. Available from : http://www.elsevier.es/es-revista-regio-revista-internacional-grupos-investigacion-339-articulo-manejo-las-ulceras-cutaneas-origen-X2253645012578954

27Martins AMO, Bandeira AR, Martins JCA. Training for wound care: the potential of simulation. IN: Malagutti W. Feridas: conceitos e actualidades. Sao Paulo: Martinari, 2015.

28Haisfield-wolfe ME, Rund C. Malignant cutaneous wounds: developing education for hospice, oncology and wound care nurses. *Int J Palliat Nurs* [Internet] 2002 Feb.
[cited 2016 Aug 28] 8(2):57-66. DOI: 10.12968/ijpn.2002.8.2.10240

29Firmino F. Patients with neoplastic wounds in Palliative Care Services: contributions to the development of nursing intervention protocols. *Rev Bras Cancerol* [Internet] 2005. [cited 2016 Aug 30] 51(4):347-59. Availabre from: http://www 1.inca. gov.br/rbc/n 51 /v04/pdf/revisao6.pdf

30Willis S, Sutton J. Managing complex palliative wounds: an interactive educational approach for district nurses. *Int J Palliat Nurs* [Internet] 2013 Sept [cited 2016 Sept 01] 19(9):457-62. DOI: 10.12968/ijpn.2013.19.9.457

31Silva KN, Nóbrega MML, Fontes WD. Data collection: the first phase of the nursing process. IN: Nóbrega MML, Silva KN. Fundamentals of nursing care. Belo Horizonte: ABEN, 2008/2009.

32Fromantin I, Watson S, Baffie A, Rivat A, Falcou MC, Kriegel I, Ingenior YR. A prospective, descriptive cohort study of malignant wound characteristics and wound care strategies in patients with breast cancer. Ostomy Wound Mange. [Internet] 2014. June. [cited 2016 Mar 31] 60(6):38-48. Available from: http://www.o- wm.com/article/prospective-descriptive-cohort-study-malignant-wound- characteristics-wound-care-strategies-patients-breast-cancer

33Dealey C. Wound care: a guide for nurses. 3ª ed. Sao Paulo. Ateneu, 2008.

34Blanck M. Diversity of dressings and coverings on the market today and their proper use on wounds. In: Dressings and wounds course. Rio de

Janeiro: Brazilian Society of Wound and Aesthetic Nursing. 2010, 58p.
35Geovanini T. Treatise on wounds and dressings. Sao Paulo: Reideel, 2014.
36Camarao RR. Wound care and dressings. In: Manual of Palliative Care/National Academy of Palliative Care. Rio de Janeiro: Diagraphic, 2009. 320 p.
37Probst S, Arber A, Faithfull. Coping with an exulcerated breast carcinoma: an interpretative phenomenological study. *J Wound Care.* [Internet] 2013 July. [cited 2016 Feb 15] 22(7):352-60. DOI: 10.12968/jowc.2013.22.7.352
38Aguiar RM, Silva GRC. Nursing Care for Neoplastic Wounds in Palliative Care. *Rev HUPE UERJ* [Internet] 2012. [cited 2016 Sept 11] 11(2):82-8. Available form: http://revista.hupe.uerj.br/detalhe artigo.asp?id=331
39Wiermann EG, Diz MP, Caponero R, Lages PSM, Araújo CZS, Bettega RTC et al. Brazilian consensus on cancer-related pain management. *Rev Bras Oncol Clín* [Internet] 2015. Oct/Dec [cited 2016 Sept 13] 10(38):132-43. Available from: http://sboc.org.br/revista-sboc/pdfs/38/artigo2.pdf
40Salvador M, Rodrigues CC, Carvalho EC. The use of relaxation for pain relief in oncology. *Rev RENE* [Internet] 2008 Jan/Mar. [cited 2016 Sept 05] 9(1):120-8. DOI: http://dx.doi.org/10.15253/rev%20rene.v9i1.5012
41Sawynok J. Topical and peripherally acting analgesics. *Pharmacol Rev* [Internet] 2003 Mar. [cited 2016 Sept 08] 55(1):1-20. DOI: 10.1124/pr.55.1.1
42Vernassiere C, Cornet C, Trechott P, Alla F, Truchetet F, Cuny JF. Study to determine the efficacy of topical morphine in painful chronic ulcers. *J Treat Wounds* [Internet] 2005. [cited 2016 Sept 11]14(6):289-93. Available from:
https://www.epistemonikos.org/pt/documents/5544ee1e20bc68f16cd9c12e2cab89d31 4d1b786
43Sacramento CJ, Reis PED, Simino GPR, Vasques CI. Management of signs and symptoms in tumor wounds: integrative review. *R Enfer Cent O Min* [Internet] 2015 Jan/Apr [cited 2016 Sept 04] 5(1):1514-27. DOI: http://dx.doi.org/10.19175/recom.v0i0.9
44National Pressure Ulcer Advisory Panel (NPUAP), European Pressure Ulcer Advisory Panel (EPUAP) and Pan Pacific Pressure Injury Alliance (PPPIA).
Prevention and Treatment of Pressure Ulcers: Quick Reference Guide. Emily Haesler (Ed.). Cambridge Media: Perth, Australia; 2014.
45Borges EL. Wounds: Ulcers of the lower limbs. Rio de Janeiro: Guanabara Koogan, 2011.
46Oliveira RAO, Nigri EL. Elastic suture in the treatment of escharotomies and fasciotomies in burn patients. *Rev Bras Queimaduras* [Internet] 2012.

[cited 2016 Sept 16] 11(2):63-6. Availabe from: http://rbqueimaduras.org.br/details/103/pt- BR/sutura-elastica-no-tratamento-de-escarotomias-e-fasciotomias-de-patientes- queimados

47Matsumoto DY, Manna MC. Hemorrhages. In: Caderno de Cuidados Paliativos do CREMESP. Coordinated by Reynaldo Ayer de Oliveira. Sao Paulo: Regional Council of Medicine of the State of Sao Paulo, 2008.

48Seaman S. Management of malignant fungating wounds in advanced cancer. *Semin Oncol Nurs* [Internet] 2006 Aug [cited 2016 Sept 23] 22(3):185-93. DOI: 10.1016/j.soncn.2006.04.006

49. Grocott P, Gethin G, Probst S. Malignant wound management in advanced illness: new insights. *Curr Opin Support Palliat Care* [Internet] 2013 Mar. [cited 2016 Sept 25] 7(1):101-5. DOI: 10.1097/SPC.0b013e32835c0482

50. Jarvis V. The range and role of palliative interventions for locally advanced breast cancer. *Curr Opin Support Palliat Care.* [Internet] 2014. Mar [cited 2016 Sept 29] 8(1):70-6. DOI: 10.1097/SPC.0000000000000029

51Harris DG, Noble SIR. Management of terminal hemorrhage in patients with advanced cancer: a systematic literature review. *J Pain Symptom Manage* [Internet] 2009 Dec [cited 2016 Oct 03] 38(6):913-27. DOI:10.1016/j.jpainsymman.2009.04.027

52Recka K, Montagnini M, Vitalle CA. Management of bleeding associated with malignant wounds. *J Palliat Med* [Internet] 2002 Aug [cited 2016 Oct 06] 15(8):952- 4. DOI: 10.1089/jpm.2011.0286

53Matute AEG, López AC, Vázquez MB, Ponce MC, León RJ, Sánchez IR.

Caring for patients with a tumor wound. *Evidentia* [internet] 2013. [cited 2016 Oct 09] 14(41):1-8. Available from: https://dialnet.unirioja.es/servlet/articulo?codigo=4625960

54Seaman S. Providing appropriate care to patients living with malignant wounds. *Today's Wound Clinic* [Internet] 2014 Nov/Dec [cited 2016 Oct 11] 8(9):6-10.

Available from: http://www.todayswoundclinic.com/articles/providing-appropriate- care-patients-living-malignant-wounds

55Pérez SL, Núñez FC, Aguilar RC, Muñoz MAT, Garcia GAF, Noci MM. Guía de Práctica Clínica para el Cuidado de Personas com Úlceras Neoplásicas. Cañadas Núñez F, Pérez Santos L (Coord). Reina Sofía University Hospital (Córdoba), Torrcárdenas Hospital Complex (Amería). Andalusian Health Service.

Council for Equality, Health and Social Policies. Jutna de Andalucia. Editories. Andalucía; 2015.

566. National Cancer Institute. Brazil. INCA Standards and Recommendations. Control of symptoms of advanced cancer in adults. *Rev*

Bras Cancerol [Internet] 2000. [cited 2016 Oct 13] 46(3):243-56. Available from: http://www.inca.gov.br/rbc/n 48/v02/pdf/condutas3.pdf

577. National Cancer Institute. Brazil. National Cancer Institute guidelines. Cancer palliative care - symptom control. *Rev Bras Cancerol* [Internet] 2002. [cited 2016 Oct 18]48(2):191-211. Available from: http://www.inca.gov.br/rbc/n 48/v02/pdf/condutas3.pdf

58Ministry of Health. Brazil. Manual de Bases Técnicas de Oncologia - SAI/SUS. Outpatient Information Systems. 17 ed. Brasilia, 2014 Feb. 120p.

59Probst S, Arber A, Trojan A, Faithfull S. Caring for a loved one with a malignant fungating wound. *Support Care Cancer* [Internet] 2012 Dec [cited 2016 Feb 17] 20(12):3065-70. D01:10.1007/s00520-012-1430-y

60Martins EAP, Meneghin P. Evaluation of three techniques for cleaning infected surgical sites using saline solution. *Cienc Cuid Saude* [Internet] 2012. [cited 2016 Oct 23] 11:204-10. DOI: http://dx.doi.org/10.4025/cienccuidsaude.v11i5.17077

61Lund-Nielsen B, Muller K, Adamsen L. Qualitative and quantitative evaluation of a new regimen for malignant wounds in women with advanced breast cancer. *J Wound Care* [Internet] 2005 Feb. [cited 2016 Mar 31] 14(2):69-73. DOI: 10.12968/jowc.2005.14.2.26736

62Maida V, Corbo M, Dolzhykov M, Ennis M, Irani S, Trozzolo L. Wounds in advanced illness: a prevalence and incidence study based on a prospective case series. *Int wound J.* [Internet] 2008 June. [cited 2016 Apr 01] 5(2):305-14. DOI: 10.1111/J.1742-481X.2007.00379.X

63Segovia D. The clinical benefits of Active Leptospermum hony in oncologic wounds. *Ostomy W Manage.* [Internet] 2010 Oct. [cited 2016 Apr 01] 56(10):14-17.
Available from: http://www.o-wm.com/files/owm/pdfs/makingprogress 0.pdf

64Ramos GHA, Crivelaro ALS, Oliveira BV, Pedruzzi PAG, Freitas RR. Orocutaneous fistula after oral cavity cancer surgery: risk factors. *Rev Col Bras* [Internet] 2010. [cited 2016 Apr 01] 37(2):89-91. Available from: http://www.scielo.br/pdf/rcbc/v37n2/a03v37n2.pdf

65Seaman S, Bates-Jensen BM. Skin disorders. Malignant wounds, fistulas, and stomas. In: Ferrell BR, Coyle N, Paice JA. Oxford Textbok of palliative nursing. 4ª ed. Oxford University Press, 2015, p.325-30.

66Probst S. Grocott P, Graham T, Gethin G. Recomendations for the care of patients with malignant fungating wounds. European Oncology Nursing Society (EONS). 1st ed. London, 2015.

67Agra G, Fernandes MA, Platel ICS, Freire MEM. Palliative care for patients with neoplastic wounds: an integrative literature review. *Rev Bras Cancerol* [Internet] 2013. [cited 2016 Apr 01] 59(1):95-104. Available from: http://www.inca.gov.br/rbc/n 59/v01/pdf/16-palliative-care-for-

patients-with-neoplastic-wounds.pdf
68Federal Nursing Council. COFEN Resolution 429/2012. Provides for the recording of professional actions in the patient's medical record, and in other nursing documents, regardless of the support medium - traditional or electronic. Available from: http://www.cofen.gov.br/resoluo-cofen-n-4292012 9263.html
69Gardona RGB, Ferracioli MM, Salomé GM, Pereira MTJ. Evaluation of the quality of nursing records of dressings. *Rev Bras Cir Plást.* [Internet] 2013. [cited 2016 Oct 26] 28(4):686-92. Available from: http://www.rbcp.org.br/details/1460/pt-BR/avaliacao-da-qualidade-dos-registros-dos- dressings-on-records-performed-by-nurses

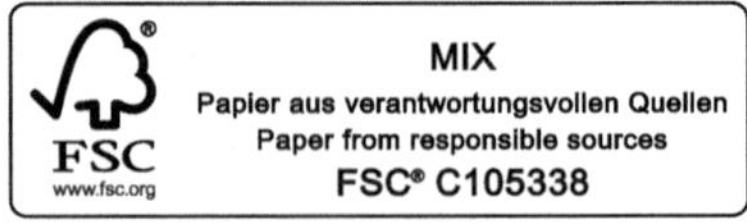

Printed by Books on Demand GmbH, Norderstedt / Germany